Gratitude Journal for kids

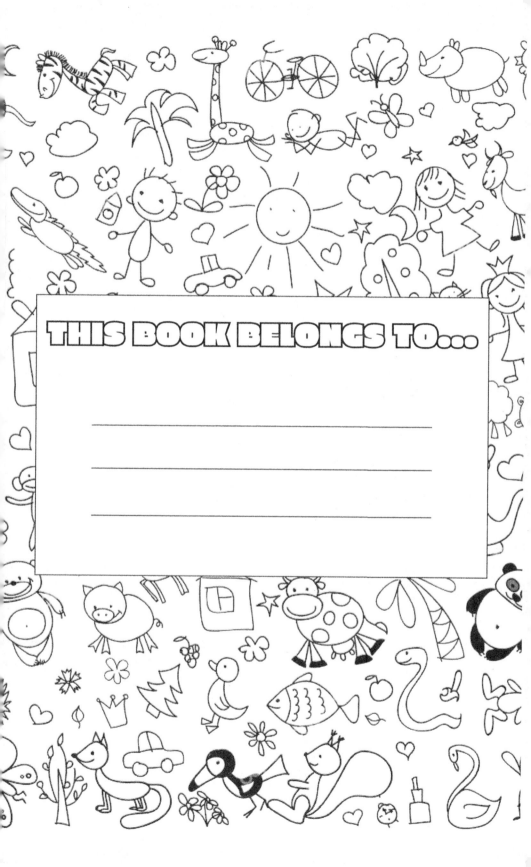

THIS BOOK BELONGS TO...

_____

_____

_____

ALL ABOUT ME

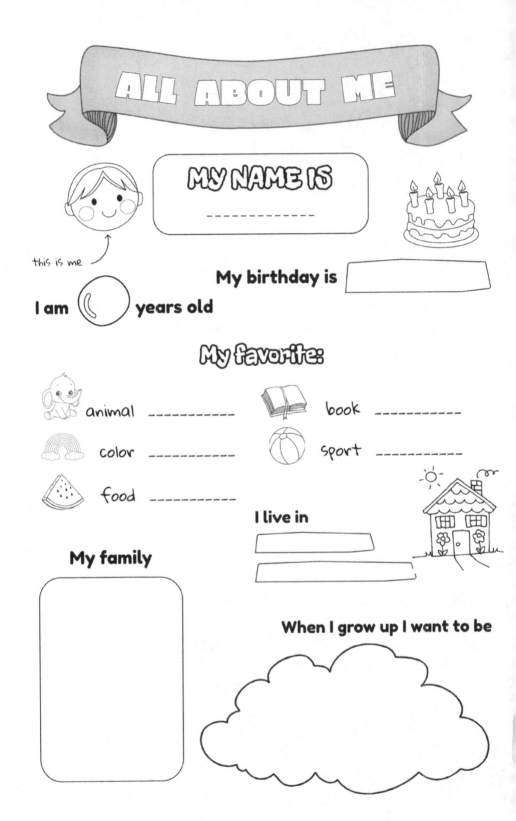

this is me

MY NAME IS

_ _ _ _ _ _ _ _ _ _

I am ( ) years old

My birthday is

My favorite:

animal _ _ _ _ _ _ _ _ _ _

color _ _ _ _ _ _ _ _ _ _

food _ _ _ _ _ _ _ _ _ _

book _ _ _ _ _ _ _ _ _ _

sport _ _ _ _ _ _ _ _ _ _

I live in

My family

When I grow up I want to be

Date [_____]

Today I'm thankful for:

1 [_____]

2 [_____]

3 [_____]

How I feel today:

HAPPY	EXCITED	TIRED	SAD
◯	◯	◯	◯

SURPRISED	MAD	LONELY	SILLY
◯	◯	◯	◯

Something wonderful will happen tomorrow:

1 _____

2 _____

3 _____

Date [   ]

Today I'm thankful for:

1 [   ]

2 [   ]

3 [   ]

How I feel today:

HAPPY   EXCITED   TIRED   SAD
○   ○   ○   ○

SURPRISED   MAD   LONELY   SILLY
○   ○   ○   ○

Something wonderful will happen tomorrow:

1 _____

2 _____

3 _____

Date

Today I'm thankful for:

1
2
3

How I feel today:

HAPPY   EXCITED   TIRED   SAD
○   ○   ○   ○

SURPRISED   MAD   LONELY   SILLY
○   ○   ○   ○

Something wonderful will happen tomorrow:

1 _____

2 _____

3 _____

Date

Today I'm thankful for:

1
2
3

How I feel today:

HAPPY   EXCITED   TIRED   SAD
○   ○   ○   ○

SURPRISED   MAD   LONELY   SILLY
○   ○   ○   ○

Something wonderful will happen tomorrow:

1 _____

2 _____

3 _____

Date [   ]

Today I'm thankful for:

1 [   ]

2 [   ]

3 [   ]

How I feel today:

HAPPY   EXCITED   TIRED   SAD
◯   ◯   ◯   ◯

SURPRISED   MAD   LONELY   SILLY
◯   ◯   ◯   ◯

Something wonderful will happen tomorrow:

1 _____

2 _____

3 _____

Date ⬡

Today I'm thankful for:

1. _____

2. _____

3. _____

How I feel today:

HAPPY	EXCITED	TIRED	SAD
◯	◯	◯	◯

SURPRISED	MAD	LONELY	SILLY
◯	◯	◯	◯

Something wonderful will happen tomorrow:

1 _____

2 _____

3 _____

Date

Today I'm thankful for:

1
2
3

How I feel today:

HAPPY   EXCITED   TIRED   SAD

○   ○   ○   ○

SURPRISED   MAD   LONELY   SILLY

○   ○   ○   ○

Something wonderful will happen tomorrow:

1 _____

2 _____

3 _____

The best things that happened to me

_____

_____

_____

_____

People I'm thankful for

_____

_____

_____

_____

I learned

_____

_____

_____

_____

Date [   ]

Today I'm thankful for:

1 [   ]

2 [   ]

3 [   ]

How I feel today:

HAPPY   EXCITED   TIRED   SAD

◯   ◯   ◯   ◯

SURPRISED   MAD   LONELY   SILLY

◯   ◯   ◯   ◯

Something wonderful will happen tomorrow:

1 _____

2 _____

3 _____

Date _____

Today I'm thankful for:

1 _____
2 _____
3 _____

How I feel today:

HAPPY ○   EXCITED ○   TIRED ○   SAD ○

SURPRISED ○   MAD ○   LONELY ○   SILLY ○

Something wonderful will happen tomorrow:

1 _____
2 _____
3 _____

Date _____

Today I'm thankful for:

1 _____

2 _____

3 _____

How I feel today:

HAPPY ◯   EXCITED ◯   TIRED ◯   SAD ◯

SURPRISED ◯   MAD ◯   LONELY ◯   SILLY ◯

Something wonderful will happen tomorrow:

1 _____

2 _____

3 _____

Date ⬡

Today I'm thankful for:

1 _____

2 _____

3 _____

How I feel today:

HAPPY   EXCITED   TIRED   SAD

◯   ◯   ◯   ◯

SURPRISED   MAD   LONELY   SILLY

◯   ◯   ◯   ◯

Something wonderful will happen tomorrow:

1 _____

2 _____

3 _____

Date

Today I'm thankful for:

1
2
3

How I feel today:

HAPPY   EXCITED   TIRED   SAD

◯   ◯   ◯   ◯

SURPRISED   MAD   LONELY   SILLY

◯   ◯   ◯   ◯

Something wonderful will happen tomorrow:

1 _____

2 _____

3 _____

Date ⬡

Today I'm thankful for:

1 _____

2 _____

3 _____

How I feel today:

HAPPY ⭘   EXCITED ⭘   TIRED ⭘   SAD ⭘

SURPRISED ⭘   MAD ⭘   LONELY ⭘   SILLY ⭘

Something wonderful will happen tomorrow:

1 _____

2 _____

3 _____

Date

Today I'm thankful for:

1
2
3

How I feel today:

HAPPY   EXCITED   TIRED   SAD

◯   ◯   ◯   ◯

SURPRISED   MAD   LONELY   SILLY

◯   ◯   ◯   ◯

Something wonderful will happen tomorrow:

1 _____

2 _____

3 _____

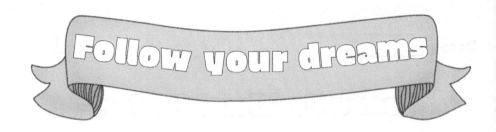
Follow your dreams

🪽I have a dream🪽 _____

_____

_____

_____

🪽I have a dream🪽 _____

_____

_____

_____

🪽I have a dream🪽 _____

_____

_____

_____

Date

Today I'm thankful for:

1
2
3

How I feel today:

HAPPY   EXCITED   TIRED   SAD

◯   ◯   ◯   ◯

SURPRISED   MAD   LONELY   SILLY

◯   ◯   ◯   ◯

Something wonderful will happen tomorrow:

1 _____

2 _____

3 _____

Date

Today I'm thankful for:

1
2
3

How I feel today:

HAPPY	EXCITED	TIRED	SAD
○	○	○	○

SURPRISED	MAD	LONELY	SILLY
○	○	○	○

Something wonderful will happen tomorrow:

1 _____

2 _____

3 _____

Date

Today I'm thankful for:

1

2

3

How I feel today:

HAPPY   EXCITED   TIRED   SAD
○   ○   ○   ○

SURPRISED   MAD   LONELY   SILLY
○   ○   ○   ○

Something wonderful will happen tomorrow:

1 _____

2 _____

3 _____

Date

Today I'm thankful for:

1
2
3

How I feel today:

| HAPPY | EXCITED | TIRED | SAD |
| ○ | ○ | ○ | ○ |

| SURPRISED | MAD | LONELY | SILLY |
| ○ | ○ | ○ | ○ |

Something wonderful will happen tomorrow:

1 _____

2 _____

3 _____

Date [   ]

Today I'm thankful for:

1 [   ]

2 [   ]

3 [   ]

How I feel today:

HAPPY	EXCITED	TIRED	SAD
◯	◯	◯	◯

SURPRISED	MAD	LONELY	SILLY
◯	◯	◯	◯

Something wonderful will happen tomorrow:

1 _____

2 _____

3 _____

Date [   ]

Today I'm thankful for:

1 [   ]

2 [   ]

3 [   ]

How I feel today:

HAPPY	EXCITED	TIRED	SAD
◯	◯	◯	◯

SURPRISED	MAD	LONELY	SILLY
◯	◯	◯	◯

Something wonderful will happen tomorrow:

1 _____

2 _____

3 _____

Date _____

Today I'm thankful for:

1 _____

2 _____

3 _____

How I feel today:

HAPPY	EXCITED	TIRED	SAD
◯	◯	◯	◯

SURPRISED	MAD	LONELY	SILLY
◯	◯	◯	◯

Something wonderful will happen tomorrow:

1 _____

2 _____

3 _____

DRAW YOUR DREAM

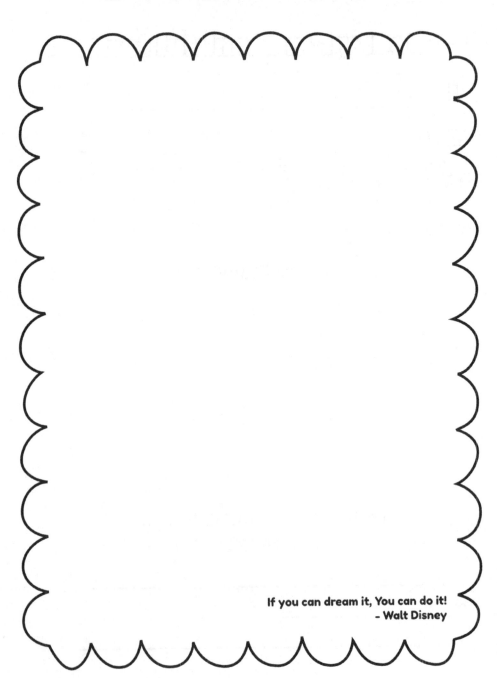

If you can dream it, You can do it!
- Walt Disney

Date [_____]

Today I'm thankful for:

1 [_____]

2 [_____]

3 [_____]

How I feel today:

HAPPY ( )   EXCITED ( )   TIRED ( )   SAD ( )

SURPRISED ( )   MAD ( )   LONELY ( )   SILLY ( )

Something wonderful will happen tomorrow:

1 _____

2 _____

3 _____

Date

Today I'm thankful for:

1
2
3

How I feel today:

HAPPY	EXCITED	TIRED	SAD
◯	◯	◯	◯

SURPRISED	MAD	LONELY	SILLY
◯	◯	◯	◯

Something wonderful will happen tomorrow:

1 _____

2 _____

3 _____

Date _____

Today I'm thankful for:

1 _____
2 _____
3 _____

How I feel today:

HAPPY	EXCITED	TIRED	SAD
◯	◯	◯	◯

SURPRISED	MAD	LONELY	SILLY
◯	◯	◯	◯

Something wonderful will happen tomorrow:

1 _____
2 _____
3 _____

Date [_____]

Today I'm thankful for:

1 [_____]

2 [_____]

3 [_____]

How I feel today:

HAPPY	EXCITED	TIRED	SAD
◯	◯	◯	◯

SURPRISED	MAD	LONELY	SILLY
◯	◯	◯	◯

Something wonderful will happen tomorrow:

1 _____

2 _____

3 _____

Date ⬡

Today I'm thankful for:

1 ⬡

2 ⬡

3 ⬡

How I feel today:

HAPPY ◯   EXCITED ◯   TIRED ◯   SAD ◯

SURPRISED ◯   MAD ◯   LONELY ◯   SILLY ◯

Something wonderful will happen tomorrow:

1 _____

2 _____

3 _____

Date [   ]

Today I'm thankful for:

1 [   ]

2 [   ]

3 [   ]

How I feel today:

| HAPPY | EXCITED | TIRED | SAD |
| ◯ | ◯ | ◯ | ◯ |

| SURPRISED | MAD | LONELY | SILLY |
| ◯ | ◯ | ◯ | ◯ |

Something wonderful will happen tomorrow:

1 _____

2 _____

3 _____

Date [   ]

Today I'm thankful for:

1 [   ]

2 [   ]

3 [   ]

How I feel today:

HAPPY	EXCITED	TIRED	SAD
◯	◯	◯	◯

SURPRISED	MAD	LONELY	SILLY
◯	◯	◯	◯

Something wonderful will happen tomorrow:

1 _____

2 _____

3 _____

The best things that happened to me

_____

_____

_____

_____

People I'm thankful for

_____

_____

_____

I learned

_____

_____

_____

_____

Date

Today I'm thankful for:

1

2

3

How I feel today:

HAPPY	EXCITED	TIRED	SAD
◯	◯	◯	◯

SURPRISED	MAD	LONELY	SILLY
◯	◯	◯	◯

Something wonderful will happen tomorrow:

1 _____

2 _____

3 _____

Date [   ]

Today I'm thankful for:

1 [   ]

2 [   ]

3 [   ]

How I feel today:

HAPPY	EXCITED	TIRED	SAD
◯	◯	◯	◯

SURPRISED	MAD	LONELY	SILLY
◯	◯	◯	◯

Something wonderful will happen tomorrow:

1 _____

2 _____

3 _____

Date

Today I'm thankful for:

1
2
3

How I feel today:

HAPPY   EXCITED   TIRED   SAD
◯   ◯   ◯   ◯

SURPRISED   MAD   LONELY   SILLY
◯   ◯   ◯   ◯

Something wonderful will happen tomorrow:

1 _____

2 _____

3 _____

Date _____

Today I'm thankful for:

1 _____

2 _____

3 _____

How I feel today:

HAPPY ◯   EXCITED ◯   TIRED ◯   SAD ◯

SURPRISED ◯   MAD ◯   LONELY ◯   SILLY ◯

Something wonderful will happen tomorrow:

1 _____

2 _____

3 _____

Date

Today I'm thankful for:

1
2
3

How I feel today:

HAPPY   EXCITED   TIRED   SAD

○   ○   ○   ○

SURPRISED   MAD   LONELY   SILLY

○   ○   ○   ○

Something wonderful will happen tomorrow:

1 _____

2 _____

3 _____

Date [   ]

Today I'm thankful for:

1 [   ]

2 [   ]

3 [   ]

How I feel today:

HAPPY   EXCITED   TIRED   SAD
○   ○   ○   ○

SURPRISED   MAD   LONELY   SILLY
○   ○   ○   ○

Something wonderful will happen tomorrow:

1 _____

2 _____

3 _____

Date

Today I'm thankful for:

1
2
3

How I feel today:

HAPPY   EXCITED   TIRED   SAD
◯   ◯   ◯   ◯

SURPRISED   MAD   LONELY   SILLY
◯   ◯   ◯   ◯

Something wonderful will happen tomorrow:

1 _____
2 _____
3 _____

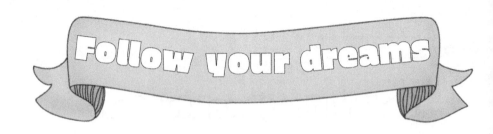
Follow your dreams

I have a dream _____

_____

_____

_____

I have a dream _____

_____

_____

_____

I have a dream _____

_____

_____

_____

Date

Today I'm thankful for:

1
2
3

How I feel today:

HAPPY   EXCITED   TIRED   SAD
○   ○   ○   ○

SURPRISED   MAD   LONELY   SILLY
○   ○   ○   ○

Something wonderful will happen tomorrow:

1 _____

2 _____

3 _____

Date [_____]

Today I'm thankful for:

1 [_____]

2 [_____]

3 [_____]

How I feel today:

HAPPY   EXCITED   TIRED   SAD

◯   ◯   ◯   ◯

SURPRISED   MAD   LONELY   SILLY

◯   ◯   ◯   ◯

Something wonderful will happen tomorrow:

1 _____

2 _____

3 _____

Date

Today I'm thankful for:

1

2

3

How I feel today:

HAPPY	EXCITED	TIRED	SAD
○	○	○	○

SURPRISED	MAD	LONELY	SILLY
○	○	○	○

Something wonderful will happen tomorrow:

1 _____

2 _____

3 _____

Date [   ]

Today I'm thankful for:

1 [   ]

2 [   ]

3 [   ]

How I feel today:

HAPPY   EXCITED   TIRED   SAD

◯   ◯   ◯   ◯

SURPRISED   MAD   LONELY   SILLY

◯   ◯   ◯   ◯

Something wonderful will happen tomorrow:

1 _____

2 _____

3 _____

Date

Today I'm thankful for:

1

2

3

How I feel today:

HAPPY	EXCITED	TIRED	SAD
◯	◯	◯	◯

SURPRISED	MAD	LONELY	SILLY
◯	◯	◯	◯

Something wonderful will happen tomorrow:

1 _____

2 _____

3 _____

Date _____

Today I'm thankful for:

1 _____

2 _____

3 _____

How I feel today:

HAPPY ◯   EXCITED ◯   TIRED ◯   SAD ◯

SURPRISED ◯   MAD ◯   LONELY ◯   SILLY ◯

Something wonderful will happen tomorrow:

1 _____

2 _____

3 _____

Date

Today I'm thankful for:

1

2

3

How I feel today:

HAPPY   EXCITED   TIRED   SAD

◯   ◯   ◯   ◯

SURPRISED   MAD   LONELY   SILLY

◯   ◯   ◯   ◯

Something wonderful will happen tomorrow:

1 _____

2 _____

3 _____

DRAW YOUR DREAM

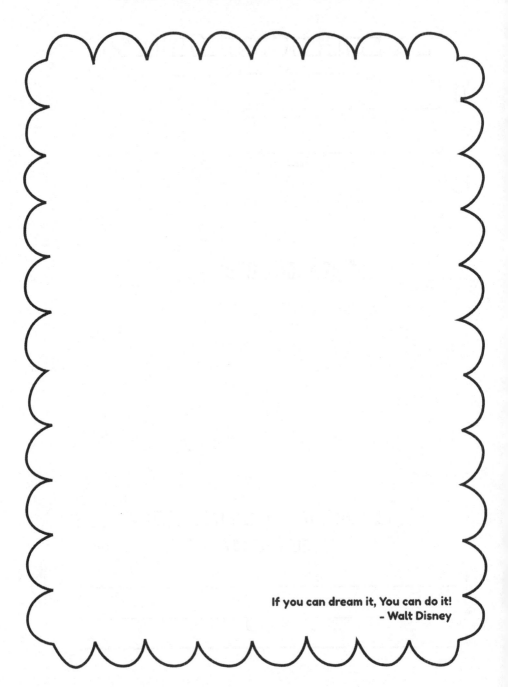

If you can dream it, You can do it!
- Walt Disney

Date

Today I'm thankful for:

1
2
3

How I feel today:

HAPPY   EXCITED   TIRED   SAD

◯   ◯   ◯   ◯

SURPRISED   MAD   LONELY   SILLY

◯   ◯   ◯   ◯

Something wonderful will happen tomorrow:

1 _____

2 _____

3 _____

Date

Today I'm thankful for:

1
2
3

How I feel today:

HAPPY	EXCITED	TIRED	SAD
◯	◯	◯	◯

SURPRISED	MAD	LONELY	SILLY
◯	◯	◯	◯

Something wonderful will happen tomorrow:

1 _____

2 _____

3 _____

Date

Today I'm thankful for:

1

2

3

How I feel today:

HAPPY   EXCITED   TIRED   SAD

◯   ◯   ◯   ◯

SURPRISED   MAD   LONELY   SILLY

◯   ◯   ◯   ◯

Something wonderful will happen tomorrow:

1 _____

2 _____

3 _____

Date

Today I'm thankful for:

1

2

3

How I feel today:

HAPPY   EXCITED   TIRED   SAD

◯   ◯   ◯   ◯

SURPRISED   MAD   LONELY   SILLY

◯   ◯   ◯   ◯

Something wonderful will happen tomorrow:

1 _____

2 _____

3 _____

Date

Today I'm thankful for:

1.

2.

3.

How I feel today:

HAPPY	EXCITED	TIRED	SAD
◯	◯	◯	◯

SURPRISED	MAD	LONELY	SILLY
◯	◯	◯	◯

Something wonderful will happen tomorrow:

1 _____

2 _____

3 _____

Date [ ]

Today I'm thankful for:

1 [ ]

2 [ ]

3 [ ]

How I feel today:

HAPPY	EXCITED	TIRED	SAD
◯	◯	◯	◯

SURPRISED	MAD	LONELY	SILLY
◯	◯	◯	◯

Something wonderful will happen tomorrow:

1 _____

2 _____

3 _____

Date

Today I'm thankful for:

1

2

3

How I feel today:

HAPPY

EXCITED

TIRED

SAD

○ ○ ○ ○

SURPRISED

MAD

LONELY

SILLY

○ ○ ○ ○

Something wonderful will happen tomorrow:

1 _____

2 _____

3 _____

The best things that happened to me

_____

_____

_____

_____

People I'm thankful for

_____

_____

_____

_____

I learned

_____

_____

_____

_____

Date [   ]

Today I'm thankful for:

1 [   ]

2 [   ]

3 [   ]

How I feel today:

HAPPY   EXCITED   TIRED   SAD

◯   ◯   ◯   ◯

SURPRISED   MAD   LONELY   SILLY

◯   ◯   ◯   ◯

Something wonderful will happen tomorrow:

1 _____

2 _____

3 _____

Date

Today I'm thankful for:

1
2
3

How I feel today:

HAPPY   EXCITED   TIRED   SAD

SURPRISED   MAD   LONELY   SILLY

Something wonderful will happen tomorrow:

1 _____

2 _____

3 _____

Date [   ]

Today I'm thankful for:

1 [   ]

2 [   ]

3 [   ]

How I feel today:

HAPPY   EXCITED   TIRED   SAD

◯   ◯   ◯   ◯

SURPRISED   MAD   LONELY   SILLY

◯   ◯   ◯   ◯

Something wonderful will happen tomorrow:

1 _____

2 _____

3 _____

Date

Today I'm thankful for:

1

2

3

How I feel today:

HAPPY	EXCITED	TIRED	SAD
◯	◯	◯	◯

SURPRISED	MAD	LONELY	SILLY
◯	◯	◯	◯

Something wonderful will happen tomorrow:

1 _____

2 _____

3 _____

Date ⬡

Today I'm thankful for:

1. ⬡
2. ⬡
3. ⬡

How I feel today:

HAPPY ◯ EXCITED ◯ TIRED ◯ SAD ◯

SURPRISED ◯ MAD ◯ LONELY ◯ SILLY ◯

Something wonderful will happen tomorrow:

1 _____

2 _____

3 _____

Date _____

Today I'm thankful for:

1 _____
2 _____
3 _____

How I feel today:

HAPPY ◯   EXCITED ◯   TIRED ◯   SAD ◯

SURPRISED ◯   MAD ◯   LONELY ◯   SILLY ◯

Something wonderful will happen tomorrow:

1 _____
2 _____
3 _____

Date

Today I'm thankful for:

1
2
3

How I feel today:

HAPPY   EXCITED   TIRED   SAD

○   ○   ○   ○

SURPRISED   MAD   LONELY   SILLY

○   ○   ○   ○

Something wonderful will happen tomorrow:

1 _____

2 _____

3 _____

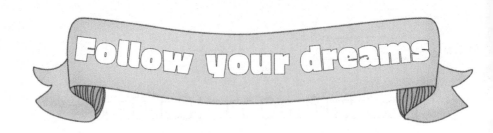
Follow your dreams

I have a dream _____
_____
_____
_____

I have a dream _____
_____
_____
_____

I have a dream _____
_____
_____
_____

Date [   ]

Today I'm thankful for:

1 [   ]

2 [   ]

3 [   ]

How I feel today:

HAPPY   EXCITED   TIRED   SAD
○   ○   ○   ○

SURPRISED   MAD   LONELY   SILLY
○   ○   ○   ○

Something wonderful will happen tomorrow:

1 _____

2 _____

3 _____

Date [　　　　　]

Today I'm thankful for:

1 [　　　　　　　　　　　　　　　　]

2 [　　　　　　　　　　　　　　　　]

3 [　　　　　　　　　　　　　　　　]

How I feel today:

HAPPY ◯   EXCITED ◯   TIRED ◯   SAD ◯

SURPRISED ◯   MAD ◯   LONELY ◯   SILLY ◯

Something wonderful will happen tomorrow:

1 _____

2 _____

3 _____

Date

Today I'm thankful for:

1

2

3

How I feel today:

HAPPY ◯   EXCITED ◯   TIRED ◯   SAD ◯

SURPRISED ◯   MAD ◯   LONELY ◯   SILLY ◯

Something wonderful will happen tomorrow:

1 _____

2 _____

3 _____

Date

Today I'm thankful for:

1
2
3

How I feel today:

HAPPY	EXCITED	TIRED	SAD
◯	◯	◯	◯

SURPRISED	MAD	LONELY	SILLY
◯	◯	◯	◯

Something wonderful will happen tomorrow:

1 _____

2 _____

3 _____

Date

Today I'm thankful for:

1
2
3

How I feel today:

HAPPY	EXCITED	TIRED	SAD
○	○	○	○

SURPRISED	MAD	LONELY	SILLY
○	○	○	○

Something wonderful will happen tomorrow:

1 _____

2 _____

3 _____

Date

Today I'm thankful for:

1
2
3

How I feel today:

HAPPY   EXCITED   TIRED   SAD
○   ○   ○   ○

SURPRISED   MAD   LONELY   SILLY
○   ○   ○   ○

Something wonderful will happen tomorrow:

1 _____

2 _____

3 _____

Date _____

Today I'm thankful for:

1 _____
2 _____
3 _____

How I feel today:

HAPPY   EXCITED   TIRED   SAD

◯   ◯   ◯   ◯

SURPRISED   MAD   LONELY   SILLY

◯   ◯   ◯   ◯

Something wonderful will happen tomorrow:

1 _____
2 _____
3 _____

DRAW YOUR DREAM

If you can dream it, You can do it!
- Walt Disney

Date

Today I'm thankful for:

1.
2.
3.

How I feel today:

HAPPY   EXCITED   TIRED   SAD

○   ○   ○   ○

SURPRISED   MAD   LONELY   SILLY

○   ○   ○   ○

Something wonderful will happen tomorrow:

1 _____

2 _____

3 _____

Date

Today I'm thankful for:

1 _____

2 _____

3 _____

How I feel today:

HAPPY   EXCITED   TIRED   SAD
  ○   ○   ○   ○

SURPRISED   MAD   LONELY   SILLY
  ○   ○   ○   ○

Something wonderful will happen tomorrow:

1 _____

2 _____

3 _____

Date [   ]

Today I'm thankful for:

1 [   ]

2 [   ]

3 [   ]

How I feel today:

HAPPY   EXCITED   TIRED   SAD
( )   ( )   ( )   ( )

SURPRISED MAD   LONELY   SILLY
( )   ( )   ( )   ( )

Something wonderful will happen tomorrow:

1 _____

2 _____

3 _____

Date _____

Today I'm thankful for:

1 _____
2 _____
3 _____

How I feel today:

HAPPY ◯   EXCITED ◯   TIRED ◯   SAD ◯

SURPRISED ◯   MAD ◯   LONELY ◯   SILLY ◯

Something wonderful will happen tomorrow:

1 _____
2 _____
3 _____

Date [   ]

Today I'm thankful for:

1 [   ]

2 [   ]

3 [   ]

How I feel today:

HAPPY   EXCITED   TIRED   SAD

( )   ( )   ( )   ( )

SURPRISED   MAD   LONELY   SILLY

( )   ( )   ( )   ( )

Something wonderful will happen tomorrow:

1 _____

2 _____

3 _____

Date [ ]

Today I'm thankful for:

1 [ ]

2 [ ]

3 [ ]

How I feel today:

HAPPY	EXCITED	TIRED	SAD
◯	◯	◯	◯

SURPRISED	MAD	LONELY	SILLY
◯	◯	◯	◯

Something wonderful will happen tomorrow:

1 _____

2 _____

3 _____

Date [   ]

Today I'm thankful for:

1 [   ]

2 [   ]

3 [   ]

How I feel today:

HAPPY   EXCITED   TIRED   SAD

◯   ◯   ◯   ◯

SURPRISED   MAD   LONELY   SILLY

◯   ◯   ◯   ◯

Something wonderful will happen tomorrow:

1 _____

2 _____

3 _____

The best things that happened to me

_____

_____

_____

_____

People I'm thankful for

_____

_____

_____

_____

I learned

_____

_____

_____

_____

Date

Today I'm thankful for:

1
2
3

How I feel today:

HAPPY   EXCITED   TIRED   SAD
○   ○   ○   ○

SURPRISED   MAD   LONELY   SILLY
○   ○   ○   ○

Something wonderful will happen tomorrow:

1 _____

2 _____

3 _____

Date _____

Today I'm thankful for:

1 _____
2 _____
3 _____

How I feel today:

HAPPY ○   EXCITED ○   TIRED ○   SAD ○

SURPRISED ○   MAD ○   LONELY ○   SILLY ○

Something wonderful will happen tomorrow:

1 _____
2 _____
3 _____

Date _____

Today I'm thankful for:

1 _____

2 _____

3 _____

How I feel today:

HAPPY	EXCITED	TIRED	SAD
◯	◯	◯	◯

SURPRISED	MAD	LONELY	SILLY
◯	◯	◯	◯

Something wonderful will happen tomorrow:

1 _____

2 _____

3 _____

Date [   ]

Today I'm thankful for:

1 [   ]

2 [   ]

3 [   ]

How I feel today:

HAPPY   EXCITED   TIRED   SAD
◯   ◯   ◯   ◯

SURPRISED   MAD   LONELY   SILLY
◯   ◯   ◯   ◯

Something wonderful will happen tomorrow:

1 _____

2 _____

3 _____

Date [_____]

Today I'm thankful for:

1 [_____]

2 [_____]

3 [_____]

How I feel today:

HAPPY   EXCITED   TIRED   SAD
( )   ( )   ( )   ( )

SURPRISED   MAD   LONELY   SILLY
( )   ( )   ( )   ( )

Something wonderful will happen tomorrow:

1 _____

2 _____

3 _____

Date [   ]

Today I'm thankful for:

1 [   ]

2 [   ]

3 [   ]

How I feel today:

HAPPY   EXCITED   TIRED   SAD

◯   ◯   ◯   ◯

SURPRISED   MAD   LONELY   SILLY

◯   ◯   ◯   ◯

Something wonderful will happen tomorrow:

1 _____

2 _____

3 _____

Date _____

Today I'm thankful for:

1 _____

2 _____

3 _____

How I feel today:

HAPPY   EXCITED   TIRED   SAD

◯   ◯   ◯   ◯

SURPRISED   MAD   LONELY   SILLY

◯   ◯   ◯   ◯

Something wonderful will happen tomorrow:

1 _____

2 _____

3 _____

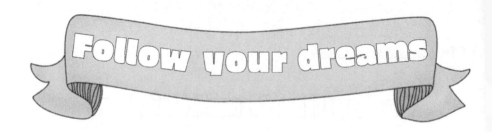
Follow your dreams

I have a dream _____
_____
_____
_____

I have a dream _____
_____
_____
_____

I have a dream _____
_____
_____
_____

Date _____

Today I'm thankful for:

1 _____
2 _____
3 _____

How I feel today:

HAPPY   EXCITED   TIRED   SAD

◯   ◯   ◯   ◯

SURPRISED   MAD   LONELY   SILLY

◯   ◯   ◯   ◯

Something wonderful will happen tomorrow:

1 _____

2 _____

3 _____

Date

Today I'm thankful for:

1

2

3

How I feel today:

HAPPY   EXCITED   TIRED   SAD

○   ○   ○   ○

SURPRISED   MAD   LONELY   SILLY

○   ○   ○   ○

Something wonderful will happen tomorrow:

1 _____

2 _____

3 _____

Date

Today I'm thankful for:

1
2
3

How I feel today:

HAPPY   EXCITED   TIRED   SAD
◯   ◯   ◯   ◯

SURPRISED   MAD   LONELY   SILLY
◯   ◯   ◯   ◯

Something wonderful will happen tomorrow:

1 _____

2 _____

3 _____

Date _____

Today I'm thankful for:

1 _____

2 _____

3 _____

How I feel today:

HAPPY   EXCITED   TIRED   SAD
  ◯   ◯   ◯   ◯

SURPRISED   MAD   LONELY   SILLY
  ◯   ◯   ◯   ◯

Something wonderful will happen tomorrow:

1 _____

2 _____

3 _____

Date [   ]

Today I'm thankful for:

1 [   ]

2 [   ]

3 [   ]

How I feel today:

HAPPY   EXCITED   TIRED   SAD

◯   ◯   ◯   ◯

SURPRISED   MAD   LONELY   SILLY

◯   ◯   ◯   ◯

Something wonderful will happen tomorrow:

1 _____

2 _____

3 _____

Date [ ]

Today I'm thankful for:

1 [ ]

2 [ ]

3 [ ]

How I feel today:

HAPPY	EXCITED	TIRED	SAD
◯	◯	◯	◯

SURPRISED	MAD	LONELY	SILLY
◯	◯	◯	◯

Something wonderful will happen tomorrow:

1 _____

2 _____

3 _____

Date

Today I'm thankful for:

1.
2.
3.

How I feel today:

HAPPY ○　　EXCITED ○　　TIRED ○　　SAD ○

SURPRISED ○　　MAD ○　　LONELY ○　　SILLY ○

Something wonderful will happen tomorrow:

1 _____

2 _____

3 _____

The best things that happened to me

_____

_____

_____

_____

People I'm thankful for

_____

_____

_____

I learned

_____

_____

_____

_____

If your kids have enjoyed this book, please consider leaving a short review on the book Amazon page.
It will help others to make an informed decision before buying my book.

Regards,
Charlie Wright